Narcissism

Understanding Narcissistic Personality Disorder

© Copyright 2019 by Charlie Mason - All rights reserved.

The following eBook is reproduced below with the goal of providing information that is as accurate and reliable as possible. Regardless, purchasing this eBook can be seen as consent to the fact that both the publisher and the author of this book are in no way experts on the topics discussed within and that any recommendations or suggestions that are made herein are for entertainment purposes only. Professionals should be consulted as needed prior to undertaking any of the action endorsed herein.

This declaration is deemed fair and valid by both the American Bar Association and the Committee of Publishers Association and is legally binding throughout the United States.

Furthermore, the transmission, duplication, or reproduction of any of the following work including specific information will be considered an illegal act irrespective of if it is done electronically or in print. This extends to creating a secondary or tertiary copy of the work or a recorded copy and is only allowed with the express written consent from the Publisher. All additional rights reserved.

The information in the following pages is broadly considered a truthful and accurate account of facts and as such, any inattention, use, or misuse of the information in question by the reader will render any resulting actions solely under their purview. There are no scenarios in which the publisher or the original author of this work can be in any fashion deemed liable for any hardship or damages that may befall them after undertaking information described herein.

Additionally, the information in the following pages is intended only for informational purposes and should thus be thought of as universal. As befitting its nature, it is presented without assurance regarding its prolonged validity or interim quality. Trademarks that are mentioned are done without written consent and can in no way be considered an endorsement from the trademark holder.

Table of Contents

BONUS: 5
Introduction 6
Chapter 1: What is Narcissism? 8
    Narcissism in Action 11
    Narcissistic Personality Disorder vs. Simple Narcissism 12
    The Difference Between Narcissistic Personality 13
Chapter 2: Narcissistic Abuse 16
Chapter 4: Identifying Narcissistic Traits in Your Partner 28
Chapter 5: Toxic Relationships vs. Healthy Ones 32
Chapter 6: Narcissism in Relationships 37
    Falling for a Narcissist 38
Chapter 7: The Different Types of Narcissists 41
    A Spectrum of Narcissism 41
    Classic Narcissists 42
    Frail or Fragile Narcissists 42
    Extreme or "Malignant" Narcissists 43
        The knowledge-based narcissist 43
        The achievement-based narcissist 43
        The seduction-based narcissist 43
        The cruel narcissist 44
        The revenge-based narcissist 44
    Covert vs. Overt, Cerebral vs. Somatic 44
Chapter 8: Narcissism in Families 46
Chapter 9: Abuse Checklist 48
Chapter 10: How to Take Control of Your Life 55
BONUS: 66

BONUS:

As a way of saying thank you for purchasing my book, please use your link below to claim your free ebook

I have laid down Top 10 Tips Guide for you to Overcoming Obsessions and Compulsions Using Mindfulness

https://bit.ly/2TDMNkn

You can also share your link with your friends and families whom you think that can benefit from the guide or you can forward them the link as a gift!

Introduction

Congratulations on downloading Narcissism: Understanding Narcissistic Personality Disorder and thank you for doing so.

The following chapters will discuss the very real danger of getting close to a narcissist. Currently, narcissism is such a popular buzzword that it can be difficult to discern "narcissistic traits" from actual malignant narcissism. Almost everyone knows somebody who displays traits of arrogance, selfishness, and who loves to be in the spotlight — but how do you know if you're actually face to face with a narcissist?

We will discuss the various tactics and techniques the narcissist employs to keep their victims subdued and under control, and never really knowing what's reality and what's an illusion. Terms such as *gaslighting, projection, misrepresentation and sweeping generalization, and freezing out* will be discussed as well.

We will cover the dynamics of a narcissistic family and how such a structure can be at its heart the most devastating environment for children to be raised in. It is important to know how to protect yourself and your loved ones should you find yourself in a tug of war with a narcissist — be it a family member, spouse, or parent. Once you recognize the signs of narcissism in the family dynamic, you can take steps to get yourself and your loved ones to safer shores and begin the healing process as well.

This book will reveal to you the different types of narcissists and discuss theories about how narcissism might come to be in an individual. It will also detail emotional abuse and show the comparisons between a healthy relationship and a toxic one. It will break down the process of healing from emotional abuse, and what to expect when you're trying to separate yourself from a narcissist's tangled web.

There are plenty of books on this subject on the market, thanks again for choosing this one! Every effort was made to ensure it is full of as much useful information as possible, please enjoy!

Chapter 1: What is Narcissism?

Narcissism is a fairly popular word right now. Countless self-help gurus, social media groups, memes pages, HuffPost, and Buzzfeed articles tell us what to look out for if we cross paths with these alleged selfie-addicted, self-important, prideful, boastful monsters. But is taking a selfie an indication of something more sinister under the surface, or have we all become victim to the hype, seeing monsters in every shadow?

My father once said to me that it's okay to be selfish. He was not, in fact, a narcissist.

He explained that he was looking at the word from a unique definition (and one that you won't find in the dictionary). He explained that to be concerned about one's self, to put one's self first in most situations isn't necessarily a bad thing. This is where we stop and take a look at what narcissism actually is, by first examining what narcissism *isn't*.

Let's take teenagers for example. You'd be hard-pressed to get the average teenager to look beyond themselves in many situations. They're obsessed with their outer appearance and what others' opinions of them are. They're locked into an intense chrysalis state of finding out who they are and that takes a lot of self-examination. It's hard to see the world around you when you're staring at the mirror all the time.

However, take that average teenager—when they're not angling their cell phone for another selfie—and put them in a position where someone is in obvious distress, right in front of them. They may not know what to do or say, they may not know how to act or even how to help, but even if they did nothing at all, if you were to ask them about the moment, later on, odds are you'd get a response

8

that proved at the very least, the teenager felt empathy towards the person in peril.

This is where self-absorption and narcissism part ways because the narcissist cannot feel empathy, towards anyone, under any circumstances.

How does one become a narcissist? What happens to a person, and when, that suddenly robs them of empathy—a trait directly tied to our humanity? Several factors, some of which occur in a child's formative years, can contribute to the development of narcissism. Genetics and abnormalities of the brain structure can contribute to narcissism. Also, the dynamics of a childhood home can hinder the growth of empathy, such as psychologically unhealthy parenting. Before you wonder if you've marked your own kid for a future of narcissism, remember this: all parents make mistakes and no parent is perfect. However, the odds are very good that throughout your relationship with your child or children, you've displayed empathy for them, and in doing so, taught them the valuable, essential lesson that empathy connects us all.

A narcissist didn't necessarily get that important lesson, however.

Perhaps their parents raised them within an overabundance of false praise. While children *need* praise to thrive, an environment in which they can literally never do wrong is incredibly toxic for them and leads to an inflated sense of self-importance. The art of being humble is essential for self-growth, for connection to others, even for greater self-confidence. Imagine a child who believes he is perfect encountering his first critic. For a narcissist, criticism is unacceptable and often triggers episodes of rage or revenge.

In rare cases, narcissism can sprout as self-defense against an abundance of cruelty during childhood — in essence, exposure to narcissism breeds more narcissism.

Whichever the case, when a parental figure is completely out of tune with their child's reality, that figure teaches the child again and again that the child's reality does not exist. Narcissists do not feel love for themselves, they can't produce self-joy. The formation of self-regard, self-esteem, self-care was completely absent while their growing brains learned again and again that the only way towards satisfaction in life was through the manipulation of others, and this milking of others' experiences is called narcissistic supply.

A narcissist will keep one or more victims (hosts we can even call them, as the narcissist will use these people just like a parasite) nearby, installing themselves in the victims' lives quickly, and with great promises of connection, respect, and most importantly, admiration. The narcissist knows how to lie because he's been lied to his entire life by those who were supposed to protect him, and he can be quite charming when it means adding to his supply.

The narcissist will manipulate those in his supply to provide him with entertainment, with encouragement, with a basic, primal distraction that keeps him from looking inward—because if he looks inward, he's basically looking at emptiness, at the void.

Those particularly vulnerable to the narcissist's behaviors are those who naturally feel the greatest amount of empathy, called *empaths* by many. Because these people make it so much easier for the narcissist to project, they're the number one target.

All the while, the narcissist is manipulating the people closest to him, he's completely unaware that he's doing so. The need to feed off of others' distress is so ingrained, so subconscious, that to suggest anything other than the ordinary to him is to trigger even more defensive measures. Breaking free from a narcissist will involve a lot of threats, a lot of sabotage, and more than one backpedaling as the narcissist tried to rebuild that connection —

after all, if he loses a connection, it means he's failed, and since it's impossible for him to fail, he must try to regain everything he's lost, at any cost.

The tools in a narcissist's kit include such things as *gaslighting, redirection, projection, distortion,* along with a talent for acting that would land anyone an Oscar in a supporting role. The narcissist has watched people display actual empathy and concern and knows how to mimic it when the going gets tough. That doesn't change the fact that they've no idea how to actually feel these things; one might as well ask a fish what it's like to breathe air.

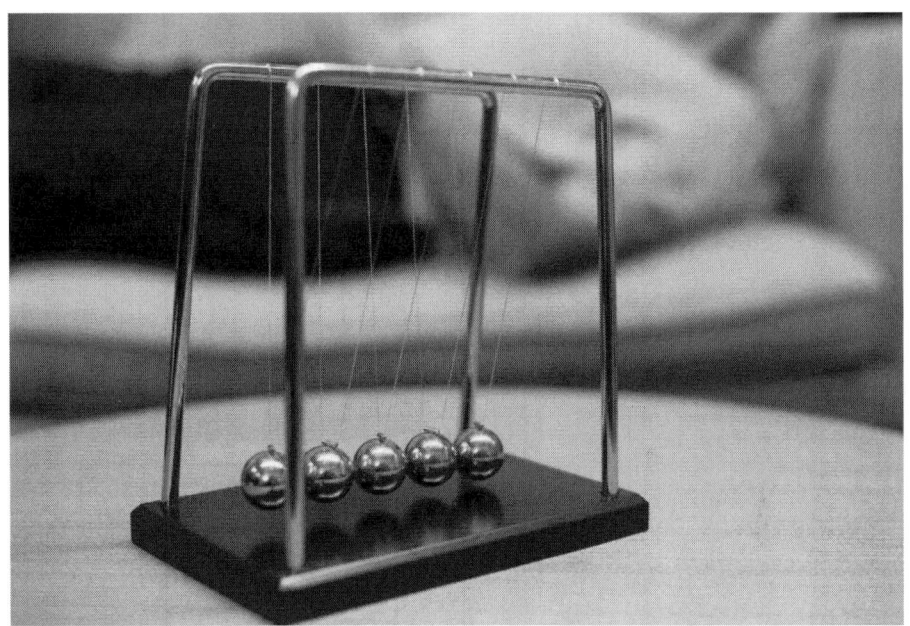

Narcissism in Action

A simplified way to look at narcissism is to understand that at its core, a narcissist has problems listening to others. We're not talking about attention deficit issues here—a narcissist hears words, sure, but as they pass from the speaker's mouth to the narcissist's ears, they get translated into: *I'm ignoring you. I'm boring you. I'm wasting your time. I'm undermining your importance.*

This, of course, is unacceptable, because the narcissist is the most important thing in the world, to themselves.

One can quickly see the charming facade of the narcissist crumble into anger, even contempt, if the person they're listening to is saying anything they don't like, or find boring—or heaven forbid, is any type of criticism whatsoever of the narcissist. That becomes a direct attack.

In addition, that lack of empathy translates into a brutal way of dealing with those close to the narcissist. Constant sarcasm wears their loved ones down, eroding self-esteem and self-confidence. The narcissist will play games of happy-and-hateful, where one moment the narcissist is overjoyed at their victim's companionship and company, then the next, vanishes, gives the silent treatment, or unloads a barrage of violent, abusive behavior as an expression of displeasure.

Narcissistic Personality Disorder vs. Simple Narcissism

It can be difficult to discern the differences between average, run-of-the-mill narcissism and actual NPD, which is classified as a mental illness.

Narcissism as a personality trait is fairly widespread. Arrogance, boastfulness, overinflated sense of importance can be seen in our society from CEOs of top corporations to politics to athletics and celebrities. All of this trickles down to the everyday person; if it works for the wildly-successful, why not the guy next door?

The difference is when narcissistic traits become deficiencies or impairments. When an individual has trouble dealing with others when they have trouble navigating their own emotional landscape, when they have difficulty maintaining healthy relationships or even being able to discern what a healthy relationship *is*, that's when an average narcissistic personality crosses the border towards actual mental illness.

Generally, psychologists agree that this more extreme type of narcissism isn't caused or triggered by substance abuse, external factors, or environment. It comes within and grows more malignant each day.

The Difference Between Narcissistic Personality Disorder and Borderline Personality Disorder

These two disorders are often mistaken for one another but there are major differences that tell them apart. First, Borderline Personality Disorder, or BPD, comes as a direct result of a person's environment, particularly at a young age. Repeated trauma through abuse or tumultuous, anger-centered family dynamics can over time result in a person developing patterns of behavior as a defense mechanism against future disruption. These patterns of behavior are what mark the classic picture of someone suffering from BPD.

Those with BPD often have tremendous abandonment issues, stemming from lack of connection or outright abandonment as a child. They believe every partner will leave them. Some even have trouble saying goodbye to a partner as that partner heads out the door to work. They will lash out, act out, and even strike out to hurt loved ones when the fear of being hurt themselves becomes too much. Ironically, they often push people away or flee from relationships because of this same abandonment fear.

The difference between someone with BPD and someone with NPD, however, is that the person suffering from BPD will feel actual remorse and shame for their behaviors. They can become aware of their cycles of hurt, and even take steps to break those cycles down so that they can better control their reactive behavior. Over time, a person with BPD can even "age out" of symptomatic behavior, becoming someone who's no longer a slave to their own fears of abandonment and abuse.

A person with NPD however simply cannot perceive the consequences of their behavior in terms of harming someone else. Empathy is not there. They know *what* will hurt someone, and they will utilize that knowledge to get what they want, and feel no remorse whatsoever about making those choices. There are many who say because of this, true NPD can never be cured or aged out of.

Those with Narcissistic Personality Disorder also harbor extreme fears of abandonment. The way they deal with it, however, is markedly different than those who have BPD. The narcissist strives to keep people close to them through systemic abuse and regular detachment from reality.

Both those with NPD and BPD have many things in common. Both operate in a sort of cycle. Those with NPD approach people first using a "charming phase", pouring on compliments and attention in an effort to woo that person into coming closer to them. Those with BPD turn this charmlike honeymoon focus inward—they "idealize" the new person, placing them on a pedestal, as if no one else in the world could possibly be compared to them.

The next phase is also similar for both. The narcissist will then begin to break down the "charmed" person's defenses and reality, using tricks and techniques we'll discuss later on in this book. That person will go from believing the narcissist was the best thing that ever happened to them, to wondering why they're still sticking around when the narcissist finds them so awful. (Clue – the narcissist finds them neither great, nor awful, but *necessary.*)

On the other hand, the person suffering from BPD will arrive at a point in time where the object of their adoration makes a mistake, and this mistake will cause the devastating phase where the person with BPD sees their perfection come crashing down. The former object of their devotion is seen through an overdramatic dark lense. They were never good, they never cared about the person, their intentions were always questionable, and so the person with BPD withdraws.

The simple ability to simultaneously hear someone else's thoughts, feelings, and concerns, while being able to express your own in an objective, non-destructive way is neither simple, nor available to those suffering from NPD and BPD—the difference is through therapy and force of will, the patient with BPD can evolve to master the ability of healthy communication and partnership. The patient with NPD cannot.

Chapter 2: Narcissistic Abuse

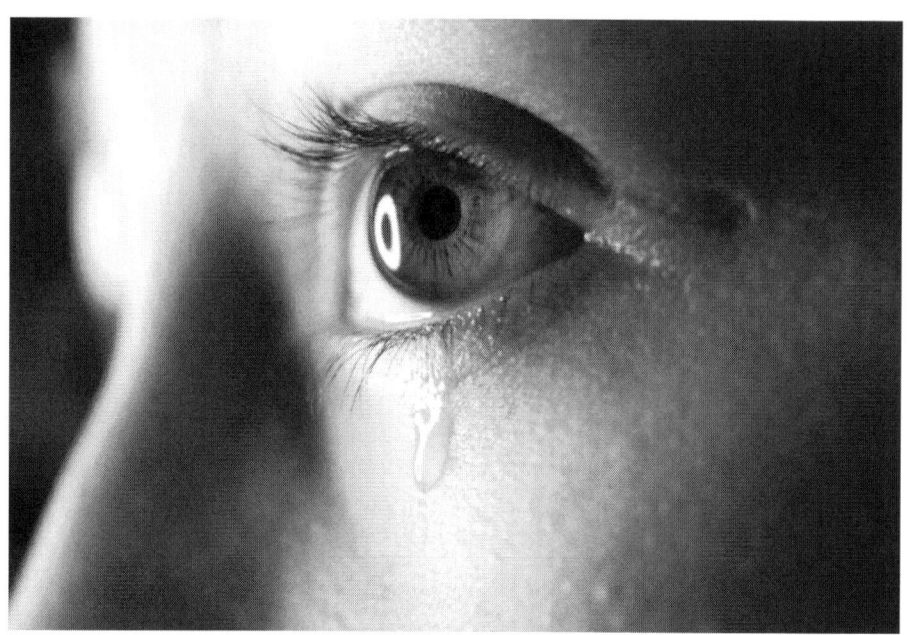

Narcissists are not typically happy people, not in the way everyone else is happy. Between their built-up, facade-like self and the reality of the deep shame, they harbor within themselves is a huge gap. They need to constantly distract themselves from the pain of this existence by abusing others and getting others' reactions from that abuse. That reaction is known as *narcissistic supply*.

They may invade your privacy. A narcissist may check your emails and your phone, look through your mail, rifle through drawers looking for secrets you've hidden from them (or, in reality, things you've just not yet decided to share with them). They may check the texts on your phone and draw irrational, overblown conclusions from them. They may search the web for things connected to your name, look at who's replied to your social media posts and pictures, as well as check out the profiles of those you're connected to on social media.

Cool hostility. You may notice that even when a narcissist says nice things to you, your hair stands on end, there's a chill in the air. Compliments, pep-talks, supportive expressions, and confessions of love, these all feel surreally incorrect, as if the narcissist had been given a script. The reality is that these words, however pretty on the outside, are really methods of manipulation. Those who've been raised in such environments are usually powerless to recognize these techniques in adult relationships.

The narcissist may neglect her loved one(s). Kids growing up with narcissistic parents will remember being left alone untended or ignored when they were injured or sick.

Withholding as punishment. The narcissist may keep money, attention, time, sex, even casual conversation (aka the silent treatment) as a means to wound their loved ones or retaliate against perceived slights or attacks.

A narcissist may exploit or take advantage of you for fun or their own needs. To a narcissist, you're not a real person and you don't matter. You exist within their inner circle in order to meet their needs, nothing more.

They may frequently compare you to themselves or others. This is important to recognize. A psychologically healthy person rarely asks for anyone to compare her to someone else because they know that everyone is unique, and there's really no such thing as being "better" or "worse" than anyone else. We all have our own unique talents, struggles, negative traits. So to be compared to other people—or the narcissist herself—regularly will wear the victim of abuse down, and complaining about it or trying to fight it will only make it worse.

It will be difficult for you to achieve personal success in any area of your life because the narcissist will take that success personally. Therefore, the narcissist will try to sabotage you in any way she can. She may lie about you to friends or try to convince you that the odds are too great for you to be successful, so you must give up. Especially when it comes to other relationships—be it with friends, coworkers, family—the narcissist will try to sabotage these as well. The closer the narcissist is to becoming the center of your world, the easier it is for her to manipulate you and gain supply from you.

Constant lying and deception help the narcissist systematically distort your sense of reality. It's hard to fight back when you don't even know who you are anymore, or even whether *you're* the one committing the abuse, as a narcissist will try to convince you.

A simple thing like playing a game, be it chess, cards, a board game, a multiplayer video game will bring out the true nature of a narcissist. They may cheat or use highly aggressive tactics that are perfectly within the rules but ensure the narcissist always wins, always comes out ahead. There is no such thing as playing for the fun of it. Every exercise and practice in daily life must serve to spotlight how better the narcissist is than everybody else. If anyone else seems as if they might win the game, the players run the risk of triggering an episode of narcissistic rage: the board swept from the table, glasses thrown against walls, guests leaving in a hurry, embarrassed and awkward, and the narcissist's partner left with a very long, hurtful evening, perhaps until dawn.

Emotional blackmail is a tactic used by narcissists to strongarm their partner into doing what the narcissist wants them to do. If the partner has finally made up their mind to end the relationship and leave, for instance, the narcissist may say that she plans on killing herself if the partner does in fact leave. The narcissist may also try to intimidate their partner or threaten them—if the partner is caught up in feelings of hurt, sadness, betrayal, hopelessness, then they are thoroughly at the whim and call of the narcissist and cannot muster the energy to properly fight back or leave.

Gaslighting will often follow or precede emotional blackmail. The term gaslighting comes from a play originally called *Angel Street* but renamed *Gas Light* when it was turned into a movie, in which one character does small things to convince their partner that they are insane, such as moving things around the house and denying conversations ever happened. A narcissist will constantly deny, evade, or redirect moments of reality so that in time, their partner is constantly questioning themselves. One tactic partners use is to record conversations, but this too will often trigger an episode of narcissistic rage. The narcissist must never be confronted with their own behavior; they are incapable of taking the blame for someone else's pain.

Other reasons a narcissist will gaslight is to make their partner feel incompetent or even afflicted with a personality disorder themselves. Every accusation or observation, no matter how diplomatically expressed or how objective, will be turned right around and used, eventually to accuse the accuser.

Tactics to keep you grounded in your reality under a direct gaslighting assault include writing things down, sharing the moments with trustable friends, and even posting moments on social media, as long as they're away from the narcissist's prying eyes. Remember, you will never be able to prove yourself to the narcissist—what you're trying to do is prove to *yourself* that these moments happened so that you remain firm in your reality.

Sarcasm is the language spoken most by narcissists. There will never be an honest compliment or observation without a darker tone of sarcasm woven through it. The partner of the narcissist must never feel safe, never feel confident, never feel good enough—even though in the charming period, they might have been told: "I chose you because you were worthy". Now that the person is a permanent fixture in the narcissist's life, they're more apt to hear "of *course,* you're a good architect", with sarcasm so biting it would seem capable of cutting the skin.

Projection. This is one of the tools a narcissist uses to keep you off your feet and keep you from being able to determine reality from illusion. If you ever dare to accuse the narcissist of something—even if you're just suggesting it may be a possibility, wait for the tables to turn when the narcissist accuses you of the same thing. It may not be right away, but you will be stunned to hear your own accusations turned against you—sometimes word for word—when the projection occurs.

Misrepresentation and Sweeping Generalizations. The narcissist's arsenal is heavily peppered with the sanity-bending habit of flinging grand statements at you, such as "you're always unhappy" or "if you were a real man, you'd..." Once the narcissist has acquired a set of labels for you, she will use them to dismiss anything you have to say. Over time, these will become microaggressions, a canceling out of your individuality, your being, and your identity. You will simply become to the narcissist who they say you are.

Additionally, the narcissist will respond to your statements or questions with ridiculous statements of their own. If during a conversation about college years, you admit that you've finally become happy with yourself, your narcissistic partner might suddenly counter, "So now you're perfect?" or even more incomprehensibly, "So, I guess I'm a piece of garbage then." There is no connecting the dots in a conversation with a narcissist. As a rule, many of them are lazy thinkers because their fragile egos cannot handle great feats of analysis. They cannot handle self-reflection because what they see, they loathe. So for them, life becomes a series of weird, blanket statements that often don't seem to fit the context of the conversation they're inserted into.

Mind-reading. Another of the narcissist's go-to tactics is believing they know you better than you know yourself (and they will use that line constantly). This is both a way to undermine your authority and sense of self, but also to shut down conversations they don't want to have.

Over things as simple as picking out a shirt at a store, if the narcissist wants to choose this moment to hurt you, they will. "You think you look good in patterns but you know it just makes you look heavy. You think you're in shape but you're not." Things such as this will often be said in front of other people to add impact to the punch.

Goal-post moving. A narcissist does not care if you're successful in life. Your success may have been one of the things that attracted the narcissist to you—either because it proved you were worthy of their company, or because it became a challenge for the narcissist to break you down, or even because it meant the narcissist got to compete with you—but once you're in a relationship with a narcissist, your success is only a challenge, a bore, and/or a threat to the narcissist's own achievements. The narcissist may pretend to be rooting for you, but once you accomplish something you've been trying to for some time, the narcissist will turn around and mention a loftier goal instead, and thoroughly erase the moment of your success in the now.

Over time, the subconscious message the narcissist is sending you is that you're not good enough and you never will be. Time and time again, you try to please your narcissistic partner, but in time, you will realize that nothing you do can change their abusive behavior. You can never win a narcissist's favor because a narcissist only favors himself.

Deeper into nonsense we go. Conversations and arguments with a narcissist often go from the sublime to the ridiculous. If you make the mistake of pointing out that your narcissistic partner should pay more attention to your children, the narcissist might bring up a mistake you made five years ago—and one that could very well have nothing to do with the conversational subject at hand. There is no rhyme nor reason in trying to reason with a narcissist. They will use whatever's at hand—everything but the proverbial kitchen sink—to disable you or dissuade you from wanting to continue to speak your peace. To a narcissist, there is never peace.

Narcissistic rage. When a narcissist perceives a slight or attack, quite often it can trigger them into something called narcissistic rage. All bets are off and all the punches are cheap here. They will resort to name-calling, threats of romantic retaliation, physical violence, threats to the family and to your belongings. Even if you back down, the punishment will continue, often cooling down to silence or abandonment for days, even weeks at a time.

In addition to name-calling, the narcissist will often begin to break down your beliefs, your identity, your faith, and your skillset, anything that is unique and personal to you so that over time you begin to feel like a sham, a phony, worthy of nothing but derision. In this state, you can't possibly pose a threat or an annoyance to a narcissist, but you can provide hours and hours of dark entertainment and ego-fuel (aka, *supply*).

Chapter 3: Narcissistic Traits and Behaviors

It can seem like an impossible if not completely daunting task to predict all of the various behaviors and traits a narcissist will display, but one thing to remember is that every one of these traits leads back to the same cause: debilitatingly low self-worth. Just like a bully was once a victim of bullying himself, so the narcissist's outrageously harmful behavior comes as a result of being treated poorly by others in his formative years, by the thoughts in his own brain, or both.

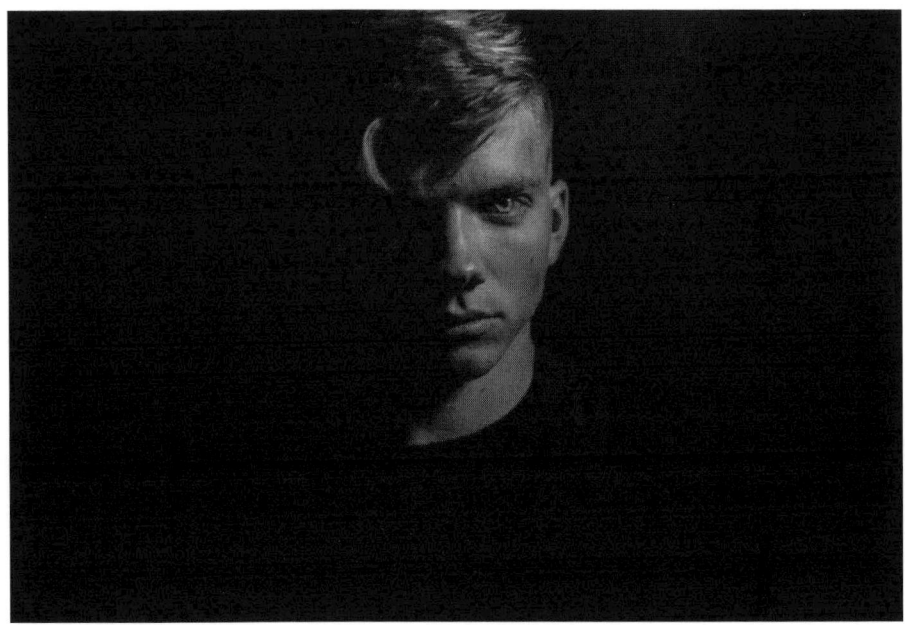

Hot and Cold. The narcissist responds to their loved one's actions with an arsenal of punishments. Some are icy, distant, others are explosive and full of rage. A simple matter of telling the story about one's day may be met with chilling disinterest from the narcissist, interrupted by a cold statement such as, "I don't want to hear it." A narcissist may attempt to interrupt a partner's unpopular opinion by saying, "Shut your mouth, now." These outrageously rude and combative statements are things that the narcissist believes are

23

within his own right to say; he is in control because he is superior—even though deep within the core of himself, he feels that he's the worst. It's the constant ping-pong of inferiority/superiority that the narcissist can never escape from, and all he can do is react, react, react when others interrupt his self-induced dream of being better than anyone else.

Other methods of intimidation include physical threats: "If you don't drop it, I'll slap you," or cold, icy stares meant to dissuade the other person from continuing whatever action or behavior has so deeply offended the narcissist.

Reality twist. When you're with a narcissist, you may find that things are going well, the conversation is happening smoothly, happily, when suddenly a moment later, you're being accused of some terrible act that you could never in your wildest dreams imagine doing, or that something from the past is suddenly your fault. It's as if you and the narcissist turned a corner and the sky instantly became black and you found yourself within the thick of a thunderstorm. The narcissist uses this quick-change tactic to throw you off your feet and confuse you, twisting your reality until, over time, you lose the energy to challenge the narcissist and just accept whatever the narcissist dictates is a reality. Some people go decades under the total control of a narcissist, and if they do finally escape, the healing process before them is a lengthy one. In essence, they have to build back their own senses, their sense of reality, their own ability to discern what's real and what's fabricated.

The narcissist is a hypocrite. Whatever rules apply to the narcissist will not apply to you. You'll have to stick to the household budget and not spend money on your own interests or hobbies, but the narcissist, of course, will give himself permission to indulge his hobbies and tastes, financially. The narcissist will allow himself to sleep in while you should be up and ready to go, or he will bully you into thinking you should do the most of the housework, because he finds clutter and mess disgusting—a double-edged sword, because he'll also punish you for the house being untidy, or talk about what a garbage heap the house is in general and anyone who would live this way is a slob. Any of your insecurities will become fair game to keep you down. If you once confided that you have self-esteem issues because of weight, the narcissist will call you fat, if you once shared the fact that you wrestled with suicidal thoughts in your teen years, the narcissist will, in the heat of an argument, tell you to kill yourself. Living with a narcissist is like living with a cobra, eventually, the snake has to sleep, but all other times, its venom is mortally dangerous.

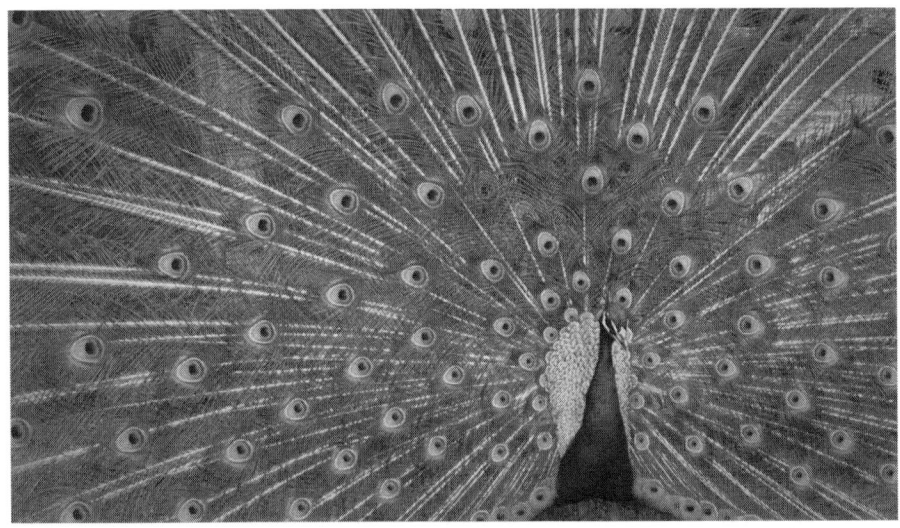

Blame shifting. Of course, not everyone is a pushover, and not everyone will take poor treatment lying down. The partner who fights back, however, is in for more extreme treatment. If that partner should lose their temper and try to call out the narcissist's abusive behavior or raise their voice, the narcissist will be quick to point out that the partner is in fact mentally ill and needs help. Perhaps at this point, the narcissist will do another reality-shift and become tender, caring, explaining to the angry partner how everything is going to be okay, they just need to get some help. Suddenly, the partner or loved one who's been enduring abuse over time, gathering facts as ammunition, going over past moments in their head to make sure they were right, is questioning all of these things, wondering if actually, they're the one causing all of the problems in the household instead.

You're the narcissist. Many have tried to help their narcissistic partners by reading books on the subject, going online, and finding self-help tests to identify narcissistic traits, reading articles on narcissism, but should any try and bring this information to the narcissist, they might find themselves being blamed for exhibiting traits of narcissism themselves. A narcissist will never submit to examination or analysis. Every word that comes out of your mouth is material to be used against you.

In addition, any shortcomings or bad habits or mental issues you yourself possess will always be trotted out as the source for your relationship's troubles. If you partied too much in college, you will be an alcoholic. If you gained twenty pounds after the birth of your child, you'll be a food addict. You may be accused of being bipolar, of having OCD, of having a borderline personality disorder—once you try to bring analysis to the table, you'll find yourself the constant subject of analysis by a very sadistic (and unlicensed) therapist, the narcissist himself.

Blatant disinterest. A narcissist feels zero guilt about refusing to engage over anything that he doesn't find interesting. If you were to bring him a newspaper article covering a best friend's art gallery opening, he might glance at the paper, then return to what he was doing, saying nothing. He doesn't feel he owes anyone his opinion if the subject isn't worthy of his interest. Long periods of silence often mark the days between a narcissist and his loved ones. He'll speak to them when he chooses to, or when he needs something, or when it's time to let them know the ways they've failed him.

Chapter 4: Identifying Narcissistic Traits in Your Partner

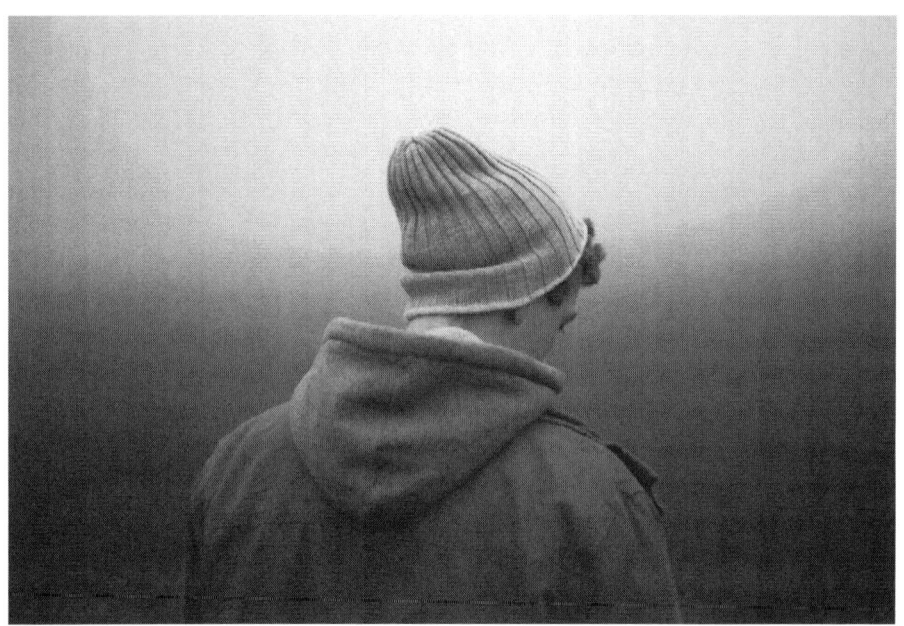

Have you been concerned that perhaps you're in a relationship with a narcissist? It's important, perhaps even life-saving, to learn the signs early before too much damage has been done. Here are some of the things to look out for and ask questions about. Make sure to start building a support network away from the partner. They can help you maintain a sense of reality while navigating the unsteady ground of being in a relationship with a narcissist.

Intractable. Your partner cannot accept that life is a compromise. There is no compromise, to them—compromising would mean accepting defeat, and a narcissist can never do that. It's their way or no way at all.

Your Biggest Competition. Some couples compete in a friendly way, especially when they share the same interests or have similar careers. Perhaps they run together and train for marathons, each trying to one-up the other in an effort to get the most out of training and endurance. This competition is never about crushing their partner in defeat; however, it's about bringing out the best in one another through loving competitiveness. Life with a narcissist is the mirror opposite of this ideal situation, sadly. The narcissistic partner will always try to be better in everything because if you top them in any area, you are insulting them.

Lack of acceptance. An important and vital part of any relationship, be it one between parent and child, one between siblings, one between two close friends, or between romantic partners, is accepting all of the various parts that create the sum being of that person. Some parts will be difficult to live with, some will be glorious. Some parts will complement aspects of the other person, but some may clash. The choice to move forward with another person in the partnership is the act of love. Unfortunately, a narcissist cannot love. She is hard-wired improperly for the emotion. You will never be accepted by her, not the good, the bad, or the ugly. You are simply there to distract her from the emptiness inside of herself.

You make things worse. Life can be full of stressful moments: illness, problems at work, bills, problems raising children. With a narcissistic partner, all of these things will be made worse by your presence, your actions, and your input. Nothing you do will be enough, and in fact, what you do and say may be blamed as the cause of many of these problems.

Hyper-criticism. Have you ever had a friend who loved to attend social functions just to bash the other people at the party? Perhaps you had a front-row seat to these secret roasts, laughing and shaking your head to every outrageous and scathing thing that person had to say about others, mocking their clothes, their appearance, their choice of partner or career. You may have felt guilty for not calling the person on their rude behavior but it was hilarious, at the time. Now, unfortunately, you're connected to someone—the narcissist—who turns that scathing eye on you and everyone else in your life, and there's nothing funny about it. Close proximity to that white-hot spotlight of criticism can feel, over time, like you're living next to a nuclear reactor.

Where is the empathy? When you take a moment and have a long, hard look at the person you believe might be a narcissist, do you see empathy? When you've tried to explain how something feels for you to them, have you seen a glimmer of understanding or disinterest? Has there ever been a moment where you truly believed that person put themselves in someone else's proverbial shoes? If not, the chances are very good that they're a narcissist or have narcissist tendencies.

Have you asked yourself, more than once, if this person loves you? You may have heard the words spoken, but have you believed them?

Hanging out with the kids. This is a tough one because let's be honest, not everyone enjoys the company of children. But even the most withdrawn person will give kids a portion of their time, especially if they're dating or living with a child's parent. And while they might not say much or particularly enjoy being present at your daughter's tea party, they instinctively know that being present, sometimes, is the right thing to do. A narcissist, however, will have no part of it, even locking themselves in a bedroom to keep away from the kids.

On the subject of kids, if you have kids, watch how they react around your partner. Does it seem as if they're always trying to win affection or attention from them? Or if you've been in this relationship for a longer amount of time, do you notice the kids keeping quiet around your partner, possibly afraid to share anything with them for fear of rejection or criticism? If your kids seem uncomfortable, especially if the relationship has lasted longer than just a few months, that could be a huge red flag that something's not right.

Others' opinions of your partner don't match up. Many of us have dated someone who's an oddball. Maybe we see the good in them where others don't. But if your friends, relatives, even acquaintances keep telling you that they got a "bad vibe" or noticed particularly negative behavior: *"I went to shake her hand and she just stared at me, then walked away,"* perhaps you should listen harder to your own instincts, too.

Lying. This is perhaps the toughest one to tackle because you have to find the strength, to be honest with yourself. Maybe your reality is already standing on shaky ground. Maybe you've already begun to question your own powers of observation. If you can remember times when your partner boldly, obviously lied, and then tried with all of their might to convince you otherwise, you need to seek help, immediately. This is one of the biggest signs you are entangled with a narcissist.

One thing that may help you keep a firm grip on reality is by writing things down or even recording conversations. Now with cell phones having the capability to record, it can be a lot easier to do this subtly without the potential narcissist realizing you're recording them. *Do not get caught.* Even if you were to play the narcissist's words back to them, the focus would always be on the betrayal of the act of recording the conversation, not the conversation itself.

Chapter 5: Toxic Relationships vs. Healthy Ones

Strong Sense of Self

You don't need to be involved with a narcissist to experience toxic love, but it helps to have a strong foundation and knowledge of what's involved with a toxic relationship, and what makes a truly healthy one.

Many people believe that the ideal partner will "complete them", and so they look for someone as if they're looking for a lost piece of themselves. This type of thinking can actually make you the perfect target for a narcissist. Your goal throughout life should be to grow as a whole, complete person—the ideal partner will not complete you because you're already 100% you, but they will compliment you.

There are two sides to the coin when it comes to a relationship: one can either continue to pursue self-growth and learning with the support and encouragement of their partner (and this should go both ways), or one can be obsessed with the relationship itself. The latter is unhealthy and leads to co-dependency, and having a mindset such as this again makes one a potential victim of a narcissist.

Stagnation

If you don't grow, are you really living your best life? Many couples will fear growth and change in their partners because it means that the relationship will also change. Change is a part of life, however, and it indicates a healthy relationship, but not when only one partner is changing. Healthy love encourages each partner to be true to themselves and their own path. Toxic love has partners trying to stay the same, like twins, so that no one ever feels left behind. This insecurity-bred tendency comes from a need for *proof* of love. Conversely, proof of healthy love is the willingness to support one's partner as they change and evolve naturally.

Individual but Together

A healthy relationship is one in which both partners feel safe pursuing their own interests and friendships outside of the partnership. The love of sports or the arts, of the outdoors or of personal pursuits aren't things that threaten the relationship's foundation, but strengthen it, as each partner has unique experiences that they can bring home to share with their loving, supportive partner. A toxic relationship, on the other hand, is one in which partners isolate themselves from the outside world, growing more reclusive and myopic, often cutting ties with family or friends as they hibernate in a claustrophobic world in which growth is impossible.

Additionally, a healthy relationship is one in which the role of leadership depends on the dynamics of each individual. Sometimes, one partner feels more comfortable with the other partner making most of the financial decisions. Other times, they make big decisions together but trade roles when smaller matters must be decided. Whatever the particular dynamic, it's based on love and trust, not power or control. A healthy partnership is one where each individual can see their own strengths and weaknesses and knows that they can rely on their partner to be strong in areas where they are not, and shame plays no role in recognizing this.

Loving What is Already True

Many people talk about how a potential partner would be a good "catch", but that they would change a few things first. Human beings are not to be molded, shaped, or trained to suit another person's ideal. That type of love will never result in a healthy relationship. In a healthy relationship, each partner loves one another for what they already are, what they were before the relationship began, and who they are growing into being with each passing day. That's not to say that problem behaviors or periods of life such as addiction, depression, problems at work or major career shifts, grieving a loss of a loved one, or injury or illness will not provide setbacks and challenges to the relationship. However, if both partners cherish who each honestly is, they can get through these challenges with a greater chance of success.

If you or your partner believe they can "fix" or "train" each other, then these are signs of toxic thinking, and they prove that the person believing they can achieve these things with a partner is not yet ready for a healthy relationship.

Detachment

Detachment is a scary issue for many people. Those suffering from Borderline Personality Disorder can find this concept particularly challenging when they are still dealing with feelings of abandonment. However, detachment is necessary to prevent stagnation and codependency. Imagine being unable to function properly if a spouse or partner is going away for a two-week business trip? In a healthy relationship, such an absence might be a challenge, and loneliness might certainly come into play, but the partner at home would still be able to go to work, take showers, eat healthy meals, and practice self-care. In a codependent relationship, the partner at home might find themselves so incapacitated by feelings of abandonment and paranoia that they could do little else but lay in bed, tortured by worry and negative thoughts.

Co-dependency leads to obsession, and obsession results in a breaking down of self: self-esteem, self-worth, self-care. The narcissist subconsciously wants such a partner. They are perfectly suited to be molded, shaped, and manipulated for the narcissist's daily exercises and whims.

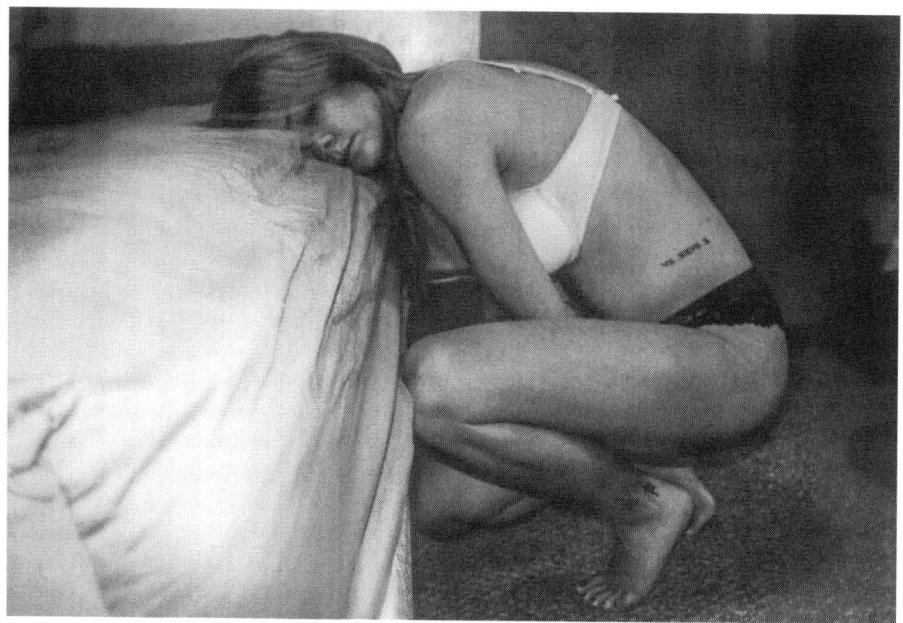

Gratification and Entitlement

Sex is often used as a tool between couples. It can be wielded as a reward, or as a means to gain affirmation. *I feel attractive and sexy because he had sex with me*, or, *I know she won't leave me as long as we're having sex on a regular basis.* These unspoken pacts made between co-dependent partner do the very opposite of strengthening the relationship; they break it down into a series of maneuvers and power-plays.

Seeking immediate gratification at the expense of one's partner is not what a healthy relationship is all about. Each partner is not there to serve the other. Every day is a choice to move forward in love with respect and loving detachment.

The Power of Being Alone

Many people cannot endure moments of solitude. Instead, they seek out their partner at all times to avoid feeling overwhelming feelings of loneliness. A healthy person, however, can find peace and healing in moments of isolation. Instead of fear, there are moments of clarity and awareness. Instead of panic, there is peace. A healthy relationship has room for each partner to go their own way from time to time, and these partners find that afterward, the reunion is that much sweeter.

Chapter 6: Narcissism in Relationships

Some narcissists are curiosity-seekers, objectifying and zeroing in on someone for a multitude of reasons that center around the future partner's unique qualities, heritage, or life choices. Perhaps these qualities have to do with race or culture or a great age difference. Perhaps they have an unusual career choice or hobby. Whatever the reason, the narcissist can quickly turn from adoring fan to the hateful, prejudiced deliverer of scorn. These relationships can be particularly painful and devastating to the narcissist's partner, as they work towards tearing down and belittling the very things that make this partner who they are. To be hated for vital aspects of yourself is something no one should have to endure.

Hate-focused narcissists are looking for a partner in crime, at first. Just like that scornful party-goer who gave you a ring-side seat to their hilarious and cruel-spirited remarks about other attendees, so this narcissus sails through life, a critic of everyone else with you by their side. In the beginning, you are this narcissist's right-hand man or woman because you're "better", you're "special", but it won't be long before you join the fray of those the narcissist deems worthy of ridicule.

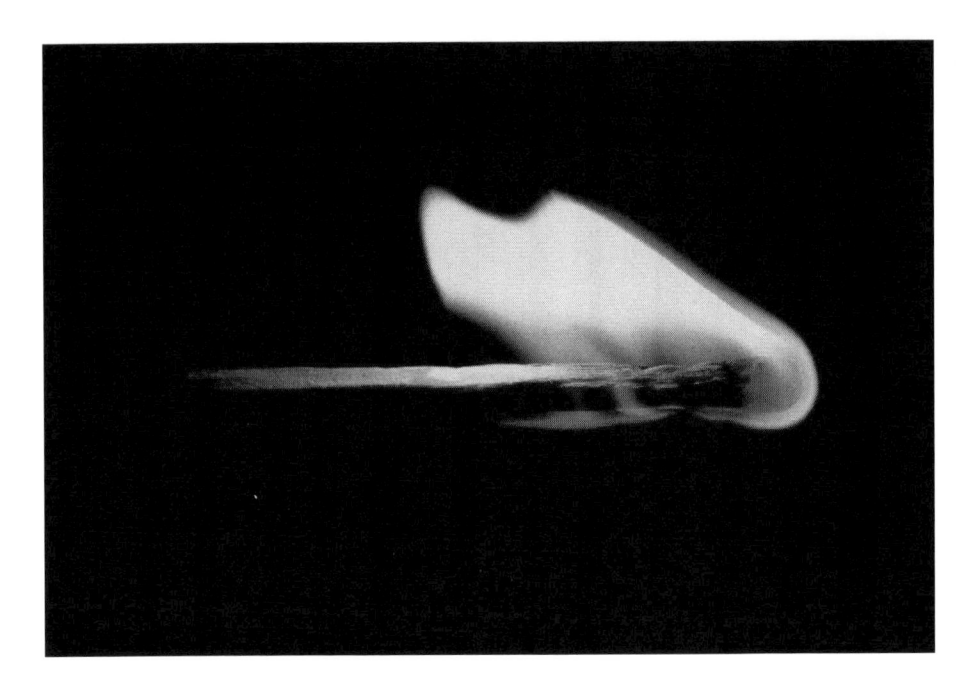

Falling for a Narcissist

Studies show that the first seven encounters you have with a narcissist will leave you impressed with how positive, polite, and charming they are. The key to understanding what you're getting into is to focus on the fact that a narcissist simply cannot keep up their social or emotional facade—it's not real, it's practiced from years of observing how other people behave, perhaps people the narcissist once envied. In a social situation, many narcissists absolutely shine, charming everyone at the party or dinner with their sensitivity and flattery. Once the event is over, however, only the narcissist's partner can see how the narcissist truly feels and may hear all about the various guests at the event and all of their faults. The same can be said of the partner themselves. Once the honeymoon period of the relationship is over, they will hear all about their own faults, every day, and several times a day.

Just like the world's fastest land animal, the cheetah cannot keep up their breathtaking speeds beyond a small amount of time, so the

38

narcissist must eventually drop that incredible charm to reveal their true selves.

A narcissist's partner has front-row seats to all sorts of terrible behavior. They'll watch the narcissist be rude to waitstaff at a restaurant, or lasciviously flirt with someone at a party right in front of them. They'll see the narcissist refuse to give up their seat on a train to an elderly person or cut to the head of a ticket line, giving no thought whatsoever to the complaints of the others who were there first. The narcissist bubble revolves around themselves and themselves alone, the rest of the world simply doesn't exist.

A narcissist will hold all of your better traits under a microscope and dissect them. To a narcissist, arrogance is sexy and kindness is pitiful because the act of treating someone other than themselves well is a sign of integral weakness. They will berate you for helping out a person in need when instead you could have been fanning the flames of their own ego. They will knock you down time and time again for just being yourself, and if you are a caring person, you will over time start to believe that *you're* the one who's a monster when it's been the narcissist all along.

Some people can become addicted to being in love with narcissists, strictly for the intensity of the beginning of the relationship and particularly those who have been raised in toxic households and have developed habits of co-dependency. These poor folks have traded real love for a brighter-than-life production. They're hooked on the intensity of the romance, the sex, the constant adoration, before the inevitable fall into darkness.

One way to coax a narcissist to reveal their true nature is to play naïve when in their presence. While a narcissist might pretend to adore confidence during the courting stage of your relationship, in fact they will react negatively to anyone who seems better than they are. If you lower yourself to them, they'll gain the overconfidence needed to start trusting you way more than they would trust anyone else. You may even get them to reveal how little they think of the rest of the world, and that's a huge red flag that they're a narcissist—even the most hateful people have at least one person they like or admire; the narcissist has none.

Never use the word "narcissist". Realize that a narcissist hates himself the most, and utterly lacks the courage or fortitude to come to grips with what he is. Not only will using psychological terms trigger narcissistic rage in the narcissist, but your words will inevitably be turned around as verbal weapons against you. If you're researching narcissism in order to better understand your relationship with one, by all means—*keep your research a secret*. Or else in a few days or weeks' time, you'll find that you're the one being labeled a narcissist.

Chapter 7: The Different Types of Narcissists

A Spectrum of Narcissism

Modern medicine and psychology, more and more, is coming to understand that the human brain is far too complex to be pigeonholed into a single category, whether it's regarding those on the autism spectrum, those with attention deficit challenges, or those with unique challenges such as learning disabilities like dyslexia or even color blindness. All of these, of course, do not inhibit a person from leading a happy, fulfilling life. In fact, some like the autism spectrum enable the person to see life from a unique vantage point, one that for certain individuals can be a boost in creative areas or even in therapeutic settings.

The spectrum of narcissism, however, is a much different category.

Classic Narcissists

These narcissists run the gamut from power-hungry workaholic to exhibitionist. They are usually highly successful in life but have no healthy relationships. The only way they can feel good about themselves is if they are in the spotlight, showing off their accomplishments and making sure no one is challenging their spot upon life's pedestal.

Frail or Fragile Narcissists

These are closeted folks, who deep inside believe they really are better than everyone else but absolutely despise being the focus of attention or in the spotlight. They can be parasitic in nature, shadowing those whose attention or accomplishments they wish were their own.

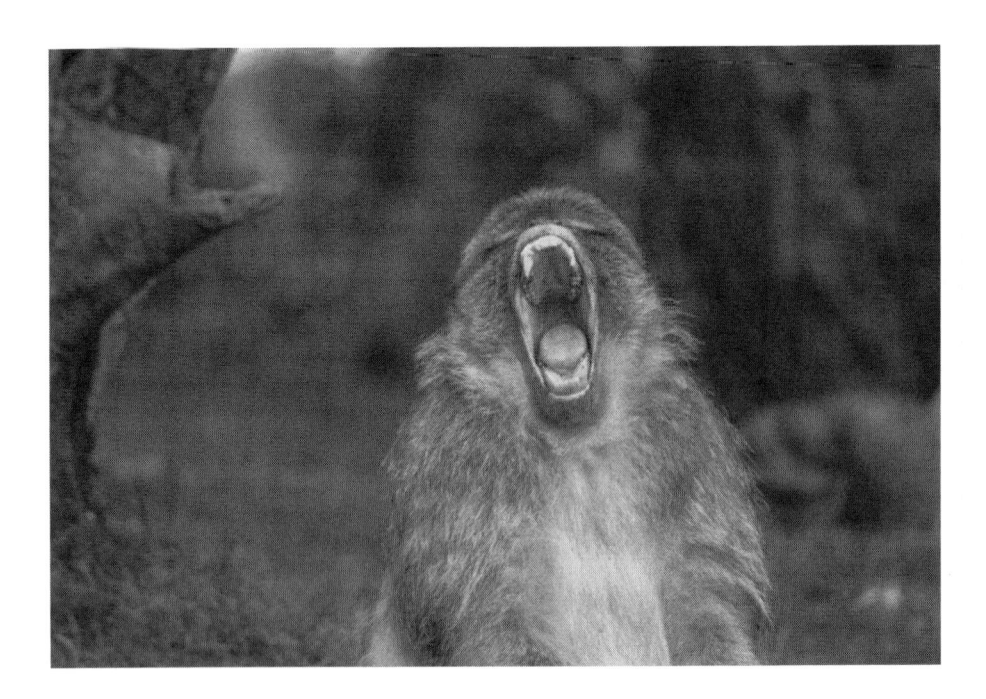

Extreme or "Malignant" Narcissists

The knowledge-based narcissist

This type of narcissist can be if handled correctly, virtually harmless. They tend to have acquired a great amount of knowledge in various specific areas and they can be avid collectors of trivia. They enjoy hearing themselves speak and have zero interest in your opinion or feedback regarding what subject they're pontificating about. As long as you pretend to listen, you'll get no direct challenge from this type of narcissist, just don't enter into a debate with them.

The achievement-based narcissist

This narcissist can be quite charming, and you may find yourself admiring their various accomplishments (which is part of what draws people into his web). He can be extremely ambitious and there may very well be actual points of pride to go along with his boastfulness. You might at first meeting think this is a terrific person to network with, but keep in mind, you are only on the planet to serve him, not the other way around. The minute you're no longer in it for him, he'll discard you.

The seduction-based narcissist

This narcissist zeroes in on any sense of neediness or low self-esteem, and floods that person with flattery, high praise, and even flirtation. This narcissist will make it seem as if she's put you on a pedestal and would do anything to be like you, but this is, of course, a ruse. She will inevitably turn the tables and her goal is for you to be her adoring fan, not the other way around.

The cruel narcissist

This narcissist gets his kicks off of sadism. In order to make himself feel as if he's better than everyone else, he'll use cruel remarks, heaping doses of sarcasm, even mean-spirited practical jokes to make his target the laughing stock of the office or family. He'll express his needs by threatening you. He is the opposite of charming. If you work with someone like this, the best way to deal with him is to act completely neutral, holding on to the firm belief in yourself and that you do not deserve abusive treatment. Any direct challenge will only escalate things and not in your favor.

The revenge-based narcissist

This narcissist can hold onto a grudge for a very long time, possibly forever. If you were once married to this person, you may find they've tried to turn your kids or family against you. They will play the victim to make you look like a monster. If you crossed paths at work, the revenge-based narcissist will try to cause you to lose the promotion, get fired, or even be accused of sexual harassment. Their ego is so fragile, and their vengeance so great, that their lives revolve entirely around plots to make their victims utterly miserable.

If you have crossed paths with this very dangerous narcissist, keep a paper trail of evidence or emails—anything that can prove to others what truly evil stuff they're made of. You may have to get a restraining order against them.

Covert vs. Overt, Cerebral vs. Somatic

The general rule of thumb here is that classic narcissists will be overt in their behaviors and fragile narcissists will always take the covert route. Extreme narcissists will employ both types of tactics to get what they want and need.

The subtype of the cerebral narcissist has them focus primarily on what they know. They're less concerned with physical appearance and tend to look down on those who care about such shallow things. The somatic narcissist, however, will be obsessed with little else. They will eternally chase youth, either by having plastic surgery or trying endless diets or by following a strict fitness regimen without missing a day. They will judge others who are less concerned with appearance quite harshly.

What all narcissists have in common is a sense of never being fully appreciated or understood. They live their lives in a constant state of wishing someone could finally see how terrific they are. A narcissist often feels like a victim himself. He will blame everyone else for his mistakes but himself.

Many narcissists will not think twice about cheating their customers or stealing from the company they work for. Whatever means they must take to serve their goals, they take. Narcissists are not givers, everything they give has a string attached to it. They are masters of illusion and it takes a good, listening ear and a watchful eye to detect them in a sea of otherwise imperfect humanity.

Finally, a newer subtype of narcissism is called the **community-based narcissist.** You will often see this person on social media because, in this modern age, that's the best forum for her. She will constantly share about the good she's doing in the world, how active she is, and how perfect her appearance as evidenced by well-staged photographs. She will think she's better than anyone else because of all the tasks she accomplishes and how much of her time she donates to others, and her ego rides on how many likes, shares, or comments she gains on her social media accounts' posts.

Chapter 8: Narcissism in Families

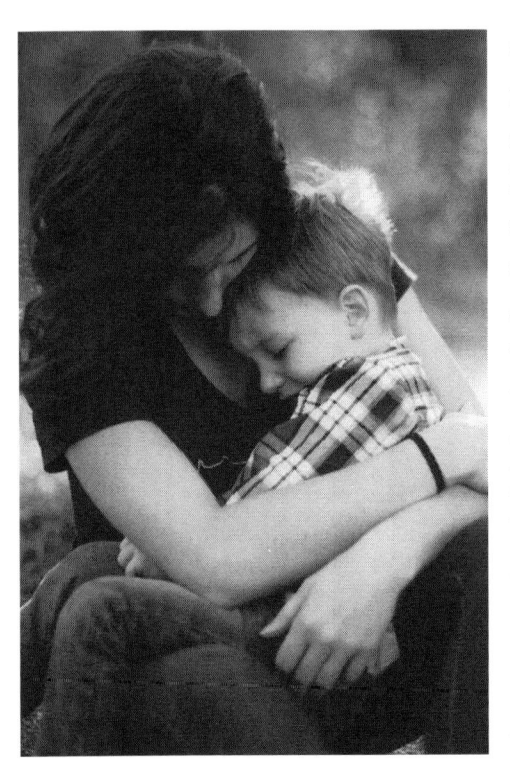

Growing up in a narcissistic family structure can be similar to living in a haunted house. One can sense that something's wrong but never see the truth from the shadows. Kids growing up with narcissism feel an underlying sense of anger and doom all of the time. They learn to not call attention to their fears however, because asking such questions is considered the same as criticizing, and a narcissistic parent must never feel that they are being criticized.

The unspoken set of rules brought down from on high by a narcissistic parent or parents (some narcissists only fall in love with other narcissists) might never be understood completely by the children growing up with them, but kids learn to obey those rules to the letter. Children surviving a narcissistic household often speak of intense, untapped anger and abandonment, deep-rooted pain and a sense of betrayal, but they can't point their finger at the cause of any of these feelings. They just know that they've always had them. Many times, they even blame themselves for them, and for not being good enough or worthy of respect or love.

Children of narcissists have to keep a secret from the rest of the world, even, perhaps their closest friends or extended family members. The secrets they may have to keep are that they are not being truly cared for emotionally, and that possibly, they are being abused in some way. They learn to always put the perfect smile on their face to hide the truth.

Children may also be fed the toxic belief that they and the rest of the family are better than everyone else—better than the neighbors, better than their friends' families, better than the other kids at school, better even than the rest of the extended family. At the same time, these children may be getting the spoken (or unspoken) message that they themselves are not good enough, not physically pretty or handsome enough, not smart enough, not capable enough, because to a narcissist, children are both competition and servants to the narcissist.

A backward family. In a narcissistic family, the parents do not care for the kids, the kids care for the parents by being commanded to show unwavering support, endless displays of love and affection, and possibly even chores around the house above and beyond what a normal child should be asked to do, since doing menial tasks may take away from the time the narcissist has to pursue his or her own goals.

Triangulation. This is a particularly cruel form of communication, where one family member sends information or a message to another family member not directly, but *through* a third family member. "Tell your father he's a piece of garbage." "Tell your sister if she keeps eating like that, people will call her fat."

When a narcissist shirks this passive-aggressive form of communication, it's because they're in a rage—direct communication is often only reserved for special occasions, such as when one of the children or the spouse of a narcissist pushes back against their treatment by the narcissist, or says or does something that the narcissist believes is a direct attack.

Chapter 9: Abuse Checklist

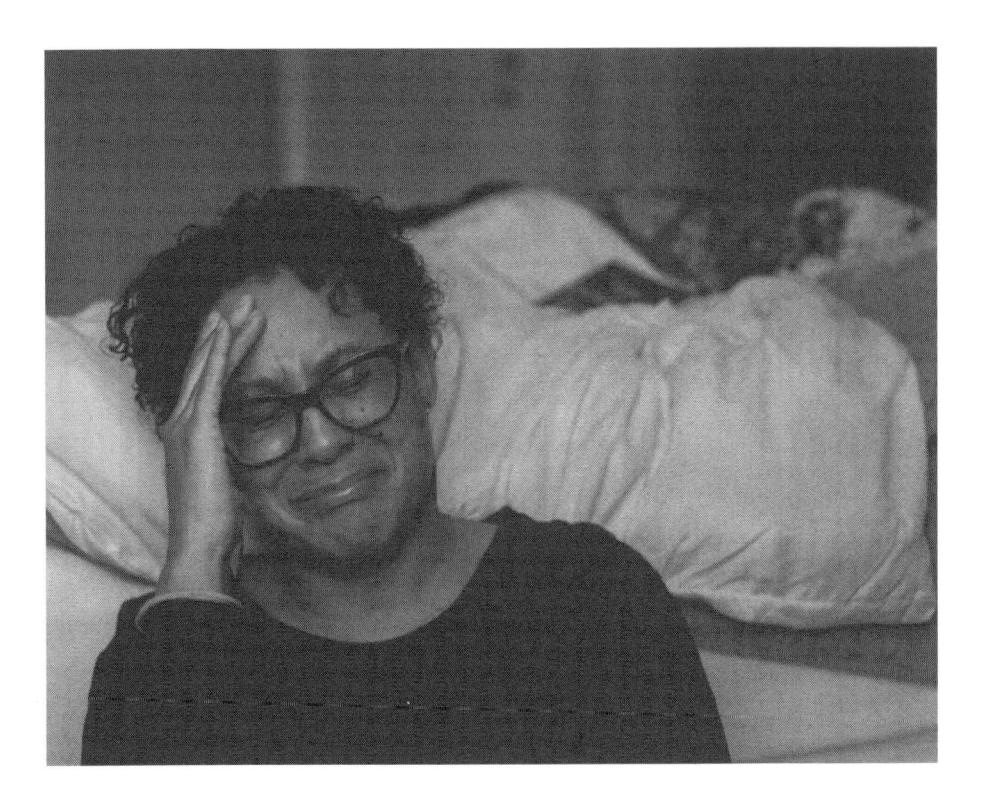

Because being connected to a narcissist slowly wears down your powers of perception, it can be difficult to take a step back and determine if you are, in fact, a victim of abuse. This list will help you recognize any symptoms or reactions that are red flags of abuse at the hands of a narcissist.

You get sick more often and feel rundown. Emotional and psychological abuse is not only a constant assault on the brain but on the body. Stress and distress trigger the release of the cortisol hormone, which in turn promotes fatigue, weight gain or weight loss, depression, and feelings of hopelessness. Excess cortisol in the body can trigger premature aging. In addition, constant, round-the-clock stress can negatively affect one's sleep cycle. If you find you are experiencing any of these symptoms, it could be due to being in a toxic relationship.

You lack the confidence that you used to have. In fact, you find that you are walking on eggshells all of the time. Instead of immediately sharing a piece of news, a happening from your day, a creative thought, or a funny joke you heard, you censor yourself, shutting down and keeping quiet for fear you'll be shut out, criticized, or punished for a perceived slight.

Your boundaries may be all but gone as well. Where once you had distinct lines that you preferred not to be crossed, now they are merely drawn in the sand and your partner walks all over them.

These new habits may now extend beyond your relationship. You may find you are more acquiescent at work as well, with less ambition, drive, and voice to speak up when your boss or coworkers push you around or overlook your efforts.

Your basic desires and needs appear to have vanished. Say your morning routine used to be making coffee, reading the newspaper or the news on your phone, going for a walk or a run with the dog before showering and getting dressed for work. Now, however, you're up early to make a full breakfast and serve your partner in bed. Maybe you have to run to the store for some minor thing that your partner has found vitally important, last minute. You've started to get to work or school late when you were always punctual before. You get to the office and find you haven't even eaten breakfast or had coffee, and you can't remember the last time you took some time for a workout.

The parts of you that are "you" are just disappearing before your eyes. There's no more you—there's only a helper, servant, or personal assistant to your partner, and your days and nights are flying by, totally consumed by the tasks your partner sets out before you.

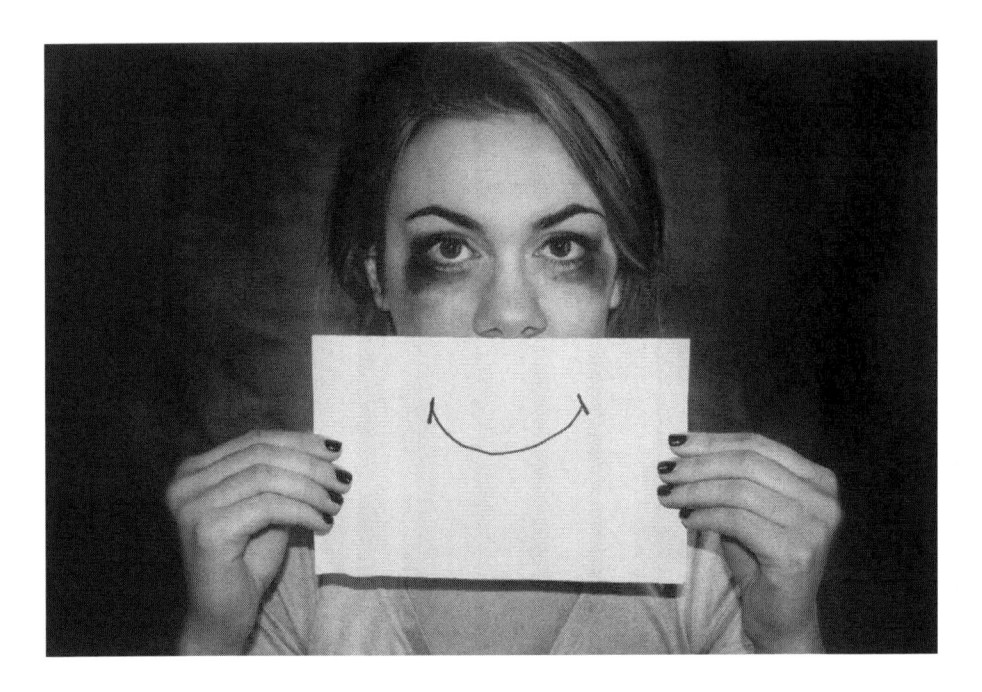

Life has become a series of emergencies and breakdowns. You and your partner planned a trip to a nearby city to visit the outlet malls and restaurants. You booked a reservation at a hotel, and the drive into town was pleasant. You passed several rest-stops and stopped at one to use the bathroom, but your partner never mentioned they were hungry or asked to stop for food.

Now you're in the hotel room, and your partner is silent. You know something bad is about to happen. When you ask what your partner wants to eat for dinner, you get more silence. Two hours have passed by and even you feel as if you're starving. Your partner begins to cry or locks themselves in the bathroom, or turns on the television and completely ignores you. If you ask "what's going on?", you might hear a response such as, "You know what's going on," if you hear anything at all. Your perfect mini-vacation has turned into another nightmare.

50

You can never tell when the next emergency is going to occur, only the narcissist knows. No matter how thoughtful you try to be, how well you try to plan, something's going to go wrong, and when it does, it will be your fault.

Sometimes it's just you that will be targeted. Perhaps you needed your partner to do something vitally important, such as drop off paperwork on a day when you couldn't leave the office or pick up your child from school when the nurse called and told you they were sick. The narcissist will use these moments as perfect opportunities to rock your world and not in a good way. They want to see you devastated as often as possible, particularly if you've been trying to keep yourself above water in the wake of their attacks.

Hypervigilance. This reaction also continues long after the victim has managed to leave their narcissistic abuser. You constantly listen for your partner's car to pull in the driveway, or you tiptoe around the apartment trying not to wake your partner in the morning. You are keeping an ear in whatever room your partner is in, particularly if you have children and they are in the same room. You listen to changes in your partner's tone of voice that might signal the next fight. Or you check your phone and email constantly to see if you've got a cryptic message from your partner—this will happen even after you've left them because narcissists like to circle back to retrieve their exes when they lack enough supply in their lives.

You are thinking about harming yourself. Maybe you've secretly begun a countdown to the day when you'll end your life. Or perhaps late at night when your partner's asleep, you stay in the bathroom behind a locked door, harming yourself. Maybe you drive to work and imagine driving into the highway median. All of this terrifies you, but the thoughts keep coming. You don't see a way out.

You are withdrawing from everyone else but your partner. Perhaps you're ashamed of the situation you've gotten yourself into, so you've stopped sharing with friends what's going on in your life. Your partner has given you backlash too many times for going out without them, but either never wants to go out as a couple, or never wants to go out with you and your friends—or, when you do go out as a group, your partner is so rude to your friends that you wish you'd never gone out in the first place. So, you stay home night after night, losing yourself to the vortex that is the suffocating dynamic between you and the partner who's running your life.

Self-sabotage. Not only are you more passive and fearful at the workplace, but in all aspects of life, you've stopped being a go-getter. Projects you began with gusto are gathering dust. Routines you started to better yourself: working out, going to therapy, yoga, gardening, are all falling by the wayside as you feel less confident, more drained, more confused day to day in which direction you should go. You might be letting deadlines pass you by, convinced you had no chance of success regardless of your initial hopes and dreams.

Disassociation. You find yourself "tuning out" in times of extreme stress, and find that you've lost time, or can't remember the exact details of a situation.

You are starting to wonder if you're the abusive one. This is perhaps the most insidious effect a narcissist has on her partner—actually convincing, over time and through such methods as projection, gaslighting, redirection, and freezing out—that they are the narcissist or mentally ill person. You start to question every move and word, wondering if you, in fact, have any empathy, at all. Maybe you only care about yourself. But if so, why would you be here serving your partner? Your partner may have already tried to convince you that you are not, in fact, serving them, but torturing them, holding them down. This devastating destruction of self is often what keeps victims with their abusive partners for years, for decades, or for life.

The truth you need to have the courage to discover is that no part of this abuse has been your fault. None of it. The strength to realize that and follow through with recovery is enormous, but if you've survived this far, you're strong enough to survive escape, and strong enough to one day begin to heal.

Chapter 10: How to Take Control of Your Life

The single most difficult thing about recovering from narcissistic abuse is the actual distancing from the narcissist. Your narcissistic partner will move heaven and Earth to try to keep you from leaving, in every unkind way imaginable, including threats, slander, destruction of property, and complicated legal battles. At times, it may seem easier to just give up and stay with your abuser, but you mustn't give up — a happier future is possible, even if the road ahead is going to be a bumpy one.

Coming to terms with a shattered belief system

There are many things you will have to work through and accept after realizing your partner is a narcissist and deciding to work towards gaining independence from the relationship. First, you will have to process that where once you believed in the goodness of humanity, now you are questioning that belief, wondering how you can ever trust anyone again after seeing what true evil looks like.

Additionally, you will be moving forward without a single happy memory to hold onto for sentimental value. Everything in the past of this relationship will be hurtful to remember. That's not easy, because even in rocky relationships, there are usually some good times to hold onto and say, "well, at least we tried." You and the narcissist were both trying, but for different ends: the narcissist tried to keep you down, and you simply tried to survive.

Steps to take before recovery can begin

Before you're even ready for the healing to begin, you're going to have to gain the mindset to move towards the healing process itself. That mindset includes some very painful lessons, including the realization and acceptance that nothing about your relationship with the narcissist was what it seemed. This can be a devastating thing to accept. You may feel shaken to your core, even shell-shocked, to use the term used commonly by veterans suffering from PTSD. Daily and nightly bouts of nonsensical, constant, and devastating abuse and reactionary rage can level the strongest person.

Once you realize that everything was a lie, the next stage of recovery can be even more exhausting. You will begin to see, either on your own through hindsight and self-realization or with the help of a therapist all the red flags you either missed or ignored going in, and throughout the rest of the relationship. At this point, you might begin to doubt your own intelligence or acuity, but you shouldn't. Victim-blaming is wrong, even when—or *especially when*—the victim is yourself.

After the feelings of grief over the loss of your own power have subsided somewhat, you may begin to feel anger, even rage, at being made a fool of. You may find that you're angry at yourself for participating in your own destruction via the narcissist's designs. Ruminating—going over past events and finding the negative aspects in them—is likely what's going to be happening now, again and again, and reliving those darkly emotional moments can be tough to do by yourself. A therapist is best to help you weather these internal storms that are necessary for you to deal with in order to move onward towards healing.

Try to avoid having internal dialogues like, *"Only an idiot would fall for that"*, or *"There must be something wrong with me that I allowed this to happen."* While it's understandable for you to be thinking these things of yourself, there is nothing helpful about these thoughts and they will bar you from any type of healing and recovery.

On the other hand, it's perfectly healthy and within your right to examine your past actions and decisions and realize the mistakes you've made, such as staying when you considered leaving, or forgiving your narcissistic partner abusive actions and words. By recognizing these mistakes, you can avoid making them again in the future. You must tell yourself "never again."

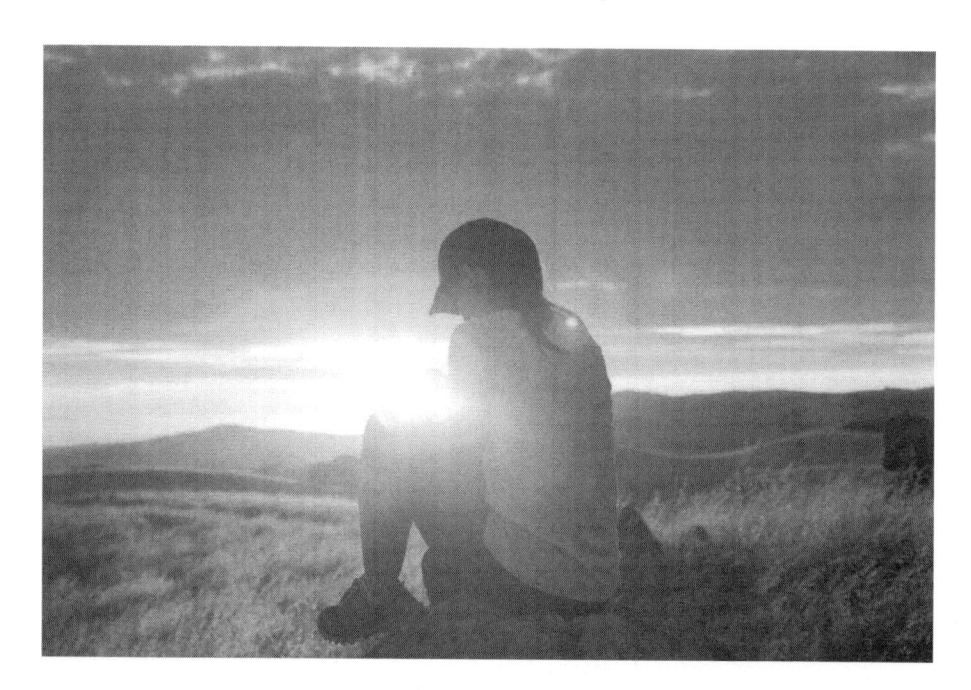

Learning to be powerful again

For a while—perhaps even a long while—after leaving a toxic relationship with a narcissist, you may go about your day on autopilot, completing tasks and doing things but never really making any decisions, never moving forward with any sense of purpose. That is because you've spent so much time without your power; no one in a constant, defense position is able to be proactive about things. Once you realize that you're now walking through life, robot-like, you can begin to take steps to regain your former strength and purpose. Make a list of small, easy things you'd like to accomplish in a week or in a month. Go at your own pace. Attach no guilt to how long it takes you. You're in training now, or rather—rehabilitation. You're re-learning how to be a purposeful, vital, strong human being.

Right now, it's your own force of will that's going to pull you through the darkness to the other side, to happiness again. It's the only thing you've got, aside from friends and family and a therapist. Unfortunately, even the most supportive people can't be inside your own head, protecting you from the false and hurtful words the narcissist has left there, like ghosts. Only *you* can fight the daily fight against these painful echoes. Believe that over time, those echoes will grow quieter, and your inner landscape will once again be a sanctuary.

Detached analysis

As you go over past events, conversations, and feelings, the healthiest method for you to employ is something called "detached" or "cool" analysis. This means you are not reliving the emotions you felt during these moments, you're only remembering these moments and observing them from afar as if they were happening to someone else, not you. It will take time and practice, but going over these events in a neutral, objective way will help you gain the learning you need from them, without carrying the burden of the difficult emotions once attached to them.

Many people use personal journals to process difficult events, but in the case of narcissistic abuse, writing can actually stir up those old, painful emotions, sending you into periods of reliving the abuse and experiencing the emotions all over again. Talk to your therapist to see what best ways you can re-tell the stories, if you need to, without re-living the pain.

The rest of the world is not narcissists

After suffering the breathtaking betrayal and grief that's involved with walking away from the aftermath of an abusive relationship with a narcissist, you should be focusing on yourself, relearning who you actually are, and remembering how to do the basic, human things you were confident about before you got swept up into the narcissist's world.

When this initial period is over, however, you may start turning your eye to the rest of the world. Obviously, it is not a good idea to rush into any new relationships, but more importantly, you should avoid believing that just because you were hurt by a narcissist, everyone else you encounter is a narcissist, too.

Now that you know what to look out for, you can see red flags immediately, remembering that the first 7 encounters with a narcissist will usually be very pleasant. Once you begin to see evidence of lack of empathy, lack of listening skills, and signs of grandiose confidence or arrogance, you can deftly maneuver away from another potentially abusive situation. The key here is to pay attention. Someone having a bad day and not being to focus on someone else's input (temporarily, perhaps their baby kept them up all night or they've been working double shifts for a week) does not imply a narcissist make. Use the vital knowledge you learned first-hand to better determine who is safe and who is not.

Believe that you deserve compassion

This is one of those moments where "faking it" until you "make it" may come in handy. You must turn the corner on self-criticism and begin to practice self-compassion. Even if you don't believe you are worthy of compassion at first, if your interior monologue is filled with such things as *it's okay, you're a good person* or *you deserve kindness*, eventually, this will become rote, and instead of feeling like an impostor who's reading lines from a script, you will believe the words you're repeating as truth.

Understand that what happened to you can happen to anyone. You are not unique in your mistakes or the fact that you were deceived by a narcissist. Some of the strongest people in the world have fallen prey to the same predators, and come out the other side to live productive, happy lives. So too, can you.

One powerful tool in post-narcissistic healing is meditation and mindfulness. Meditation often gets a bad rap as being too complicated, too New Age, having religious affiliations and being something people with a lot more time on their hands can do, not the everyday person. This all could not be farther from the truth. Meditation is nearly universal and based on tremendously simple ideas. If one takes a small amount of time each day to sit with good posture and practice deep breathing and detached thinking, one can reduce stress in the brain and in the body, prolong longevity, fight depression and anxiety, and even improve cognitive function over time. That's all there is to it.

One of the things a practitioner of meditation will do is something called "detached thinking". Thoughts will invade the mind's space, it's inevitable even with the seasoned meditator. During meditation, however, instead of allowing that invading thought to lead you away into a thorough discussion or examination, you simply mark that thought for what it is and let it drift away. *A memory of when we went to the restaurant, when she threw a plate against the wall, the night I drove to my sister's and slept on her couch.* Recognize the thoughts and memories but nothing more. Just like a child's game on a car trip to describe what they see: *bird, tree, train, house*, so are you simply marking the thoughts, and allowing them to fall away, into the calm and unbroken state of mindfulness.

When complete detachment is not an option

Many survivors of a narcissistic relationship must, unfortunately, keep in contact with their abuser because of children. This is perhaps the cruelest thing of all, and your narcissistic ex-partner will try everything in your power to use this necessary relationship to hurt you. The best thing you can do for yourself, and for the children, is to not engage and not retaliate. Over time, others will see the truth for what is: that your ex is mentally unwell and that you are not to blame for their unhappiness. If you engage your ex and continue battling, however, it may be impossible for anyone to ever determine where your ex ends and you begin—you both may seem unstable. Not only that but engaging a narcissist is like throwing gasoline on a fire. You will only incite greater backlash and pain onto yourself.

One of the methods of reaction that drives a narcissist most to rage is a completely non-emotional reaction. The silent treatment is a hurtful response, and that's not what we're talking about here. But when it's your turn to speak—either because of an email having to do with the kids, or a meeting with your divorce lawyers—do so neutrally, without hurtful language or accusatory tones. Your ex may reach higher levels of rage, but you will be able to weather it without taking any damage to your psyche or reputation.

Slow and steady (wins the race)

There might be many days when you'll wish you can just jump in your car and put thousands of miles between yourself and your former abuser, but even that wouldn't accomplish the healing you're going to need. Your narcissist would still try to seek you out, even if you moved halfway across the world from him or her.

The battles you face are going to be right in front of you, as well as inside your own mind and heart. You may have to fight these battles in front of your abuser if they co-parent with you. Because of the difficulty of this, you need to take things slowly, and have patience with yourself that in time, things are going to be all right—*you* are going to be all right.

Don't be afraid to reach out to your trusted support network if you feel you're about to take a step backward. Healing journeys are never perfect inclines; there are peaks and valleys along the way. Do not associate with anyone who shames you for still feeling pain and loss a month, a year, five years later. Everyone grieves and heals differently, and emotions should never be sources of shame.

Think about what you want in your life, and think about where you can find it today, now. Think about the people who personify these things. Surround yourself with as much positivity, gentle kindness, forgiveness, and compassion as you can. These are the best parts of being human, and they're real, they exist, and they're not weaknesses—the greatest heroes in the world practice them. There are countless zen sayings about how a gently-flowing stream can carve through the tallest, most formidable mountain, and how the tree that is able to bend in the wind cannot be broken by the wind.

The proof of this is that you are here, standing now, and you're not yet broken—not completely. You have weathered the constant storms to come out the other side, still hopeful for a happy life. Do not berate yourself for having this hope. It's the biggest sign that you are indeed, a good person, and that you're strong enough to believe in yourself and in the good in the world.

You are a hero for choosing these aspects of life and turning away from cruelty, and narcissism.

Conclusion

Thank you for making it through to the end of *Narcissism – Understanding Narcissistic Personality Disorder.* I hope it was informative and able to provide you with all of the tools you need to be safe in the face of narcissism and to break free of any toxic situations you or a loved one may find yourselves in.

Whether your narcissist is the one who's suddenly broken off the relationship, or you've decided to take the steps needed to break free and begin healing from emotional abuse, the most important thing is to get help now and start rebuilding your support network. Perhaps you've drifted away from everyone you used to know because your toxic partner systematically made it impossible to keep close ties with anyone but themselves. Now is the time to reach out, explain to people you trust (and who are not also friends with the narcissist) what happened, and take the leap of faith needed to believe that they will not blame *you* for your abuse. These next few moments can be terrifying but remember—you were strong enough to survive this, and you are strong enough to keep free of it. Do not enable yourself to return to the narcissist, no matter what. The No Contact Rule is very important because most narcissists will try to win you back by the same methods they employed to woo you in the first place: charm, flattery, attention, affection, caring. Remember that these are all facades, learned from watching healthy people express love to one another and that the narcissist is incapable of such things because deep inside, he has no self-love, only rage, only contempt, only a desire to make others bend to his wishes.

The other possibility is that your narcissist may try to strong-arm you into returning to him or her. They may threaten you with emotional blackmail, or make threats regarding your family or your children, maybe even your pet! If you have mutual financial holdings, they may threaten to sue you for the entire thing or drag you through court until you're too miserable to fight anymore. In addition to a support network and a good therapist, finding legal counsel could be crucial right now. For female victims of abuse, many agencies help with pro bono legal assistance so you can get back on your feet and start a new life.

There are now many support groups for victims of narcissistic abuse. Men, women, and children of narcissistic parents are learning that there is strength in numbers and that they are certainly not alone. Reach out until you find a community that can help you see that it was not "all in your head", and that your fears and experiences were real, not imagined. Learn how others survived their ordeal and take notes for the road ahead. No victim should have to fight alone; there are too many resources available to the victim of abuse to allow that to happen.

You might have to make sacrifices along the way on the road to healing. Often times, victims of narcissists leave impulsively, grabbing the opportunity when their strength is the highest, or when their partner isn't home. You may have belongings that you left behind. If you must retrieve these, bring a friend, or several friends. One can do the talking for you, another can coach you through the experience, effectively blocking out the narcissist's scathing words; still, another can record the moment for future proof. Do not engage the narcissist by yourself—it would be better to consider those left-behind belongings a loss than risk being coerced into returning to the relationship.

Believe that like so many others before you, you have the strength to break free from narcissistic abuse. Just taking the time to learn about narcissism and the ways it affects everyone around it was an important step in your journey, or in the journey of a loved one who's suffering. Thank you for caring enough to want something better for you and your family.

BONUS:

As a way of saying thank you for purchasing my book, please use your link below to claim your free ebook

I have laid down Top 10 Tips Guide for you to Overcoming Obsessions and Compulsions Using Mindfulness

https://bit.ly/2TDMNkn

You can also share your link with your friends and families whom you think that can benefit from the guide or you can forward them the link as a gift!

Printed in Great Britain
by Amazon